Table of Contents

Author's Note

Dear Reader,

I am thrilled to share this book with you, a journey into the world of nutrition and the concept of real fooding. Real fooding, at its heart, is about embracing a dietary philosophy that celebrates the intrinsic goodness of whole, unprocessed foods in their most natural state. It's a commitment to nourishing your body with foods that haven't been heavily refined or altered, avoiding artificial additives, preservatives, and excessive processing.

The real fooding journey is not just about what you eat; it's a profound shift in how you relate to food and the world around you. It's an invitation to reconnect with the wisdom of nature, to savor the flavors of unadulterated ingredients, and to nourish your body in a way that honors its innate needs.

In these pages, we'll delve into the richness of real fooding, exploring the benefits it brings to our health, our well-being, and the environment. I invite you to immerse yourself into the world of real fooding, and to make it a part of your daily life.

Mitxel Gonzalez.

Chapter 1: Introduction to Nutrition and Real Fooding

In this inaugural chapter, we embark on a journey into the world of nutrition and real fooding, laying the foundation for a profound understanding of how dietary choices impact our health and well-being. Let's delve into each of the three subchapters in detail.

1.1 Definition of Nutrition and Real Fooding

Definition of Nutrition

Nutrition is far more than a simple choice between what to eat and what not to eat. It is a science, a practice, and an intricate web of processes that dictate how our bodies function, grow, and thrive. At its core, nutrition is the study of how we acquire, utilize, and assimilate essential nutrients from the foods we consume.

These nutrients encompass a spectrum of vital components, from the macronutrients—carbohydrates, proteins, and fats—that provide us with energy, to the micronutrients—vitamins and minerals—that act as catalysts and regulators in countless biochemical reactions within our bodies.

The significance of nutrition extends beyond mere sustenance; it influences nearly every facet of our existence. Our physical health, emotional well-being, cognitive function, and overall vitality are intricately tied to the nutrients we ingest.

From the energy needed to fuel our daily activities to the building blocks required for cellular repair and growth, nutrition is the cornerstone upon which our lives are built.

Definition of Real Fooding

Real fooding is more than just a dietary choice; it's a philosophy, a commitment to nourishing the body and soul with foods that align with the wisdom of nature. At its essence, real fooding is about selecting foods that remain as close to their natural state as possible, unfettered by excessive processing, artificial additives, or preservatives.

In the realm of real fooding, the journey from farm to table is a simple and transparent one. It champions the consumption of ingredients that are readily recognizable, unadulterated, and brimming with essential nutrients. These are the foods that our ancestors thrived on for generations, foods that have sustained humanity for millennia.

Real fooding isn't merely a return to tradition; it's a celebration of the abundance and diversity that our planet offers. It's an acknowledgment that food is more than fuel—it's a source of pleasure, connection, and cultural richness.

In an era marked by convenience-driven consumables and highly processed products, real fooding is a deliberate choice to reclaim our culinary heritage. It's a call to embrace the simplicity and purity of whole, unprocessed foods, nurturing our bodies and fostering a deeper connection to the food we eat.

By understanding these definitions, you've laid the essential foundation for navigating the intricate world of nutrition and dietary choices. As you journey through this book, you'll uncover the principles and practices that make nutrition a dynamic and exciting field, and real fooding a rewarding and life-enriching way to nourish yourself.

1.2 History and Evolution of Nutrition

History of Nutrition

The history of nutrition is an epic narrative that spans thousands of years, rooted in the fundamental human quest for sustenance and well-being. It finds its origins in the practices of early civilizations, where our ancestors learned to forage for edible plants and hunt for the nourishment needed to survive and thrive.

As societies advanced, the dawn of agriculture marked a transformative period in human history. This agricultural revolution brought about the deliberate cultivation of crops and the domestication of animals, paving the way for the emergence of settled communities and the diversification of diets. The cultivation of grains, the taming of livestock, and the cultivation of fruits and vegetables expanded the spectrum of foods available to humanity.

In the 20th century, the field of nutrition underwent a profound metamorphosis, driven by scientific discoveries that revolutionized our understanding of human health. The identification of essential vitamins and minerals and the exploration of their roles in the body unlocked new dimensions in nutrition. The recognition that specific nutrients were vital for sustaining life and preventing deficiency-related diseases marked a pivotal moment in the history of nutrition.

The Evolution of Human Diet

The story of human nutrition is intricately intertwined with the evolution of our species. Early humans, as hunter-gatherers, relied on a diet primarily composed of foraged plants, hunted game, and seasonal delicacies. Their dietary choices were dictated by the bounty of nature and the rhythms of the seasons.

With the advent of agriculture, a seismic shift occurred in the human diet. Agricultural practices enabled the cultivation of crops like wheat, rice, and maize, as well as the domestication of animals such as cattle, chickens, and sheep.

This shift towards agriculture introduced a more plant-centric diet, with grains and legumes assuming central roles in human nutrition. It also marked the beginning of food preservation techniques, allowing societies to store surplus crops for leaner times.

In the modern era, industrialization revolutionized food production, introducing a wave of processed foods that have become ubiquitous in our diets. These processed foods, often laden with refined sugars, unhealthy fats, and artificial additives, represent a departure from the diets of our ancestors.

Recognizing the evolution of the human diet empowers individuals to make informed dietary choices grounded in an appreciation of their cultural and historical context. It invites us to explore the rich tapestry of traditional diets and the wisdom of bygone eras while navigating the complex landscape of contemporary nutrition.

As you delve deeper into this book, you'll uncover the fascinating interplay between ancient wisdom and modern science, providing you with the knowledge and insights needed to make choices that promote health, well-being, and a deeper connection to the food we consume.

1.3 Importance of Healthy Eating

Health Impact

The impact of healthy eating on our overall well-being cannot be overstated. A diet characterized by balance and rich in essential nutrients stands as a powerful fortress against the onset of chronic diseases that plague societies worldwide.

Heart disease, diabetes, certain types of cancer—these formidable adversaries can often be thwarted or mitigated through the simple act of nourishing our bodies with the right foods. Healthy eating bolsters the immune system, providing our bodies with the defenses needed to fend off infections and ailments.

Healthy eating is not solely the domain of adults. It plays a pivotal role in the growth and development of children, providing them with the building blocks necessary for physical and cognitive maturation. For adults, it is the cornerstone of maintaining a healthy weight and robust energy levels, enabling us to lead vibrant, active lives.

Social and Environmental Effects

The impact of our dietary choices extends far beyond our individual health. It ripples through society and reverberates in the environment. The production of food carries substantial environmental consequences, including the utilization of precious resources, the emission of greenhouse gases, and the depletion of ecological diversity.

However, we are not passive observers in this equation. Through conscientious dietary choices, each of us can play a role in promoting sustainability and reducing our environmental footprint.

Simple actions like reducing food waste, selecting locally sourced and seasonal foods, and advocating for ethical and eco-friendly agricultural practices can contribute to a healthier planet for future generations.

Quality of Life

Healthy eating does not only extend the quantity of our years but enhances the quality of our lives. A nutritionally sound diet has the power to uplift our mood, sharpen our cognitive acuity, and bolster our mental well-being. It endows us with physical vitality, granting us the capacity to engage in our daily activities with ease and to savor an active, fulfilling existence.

Moreover, the profound recognition of the imperative of healthy eating serves as a catalyst. It motivates individuals to make enlightened dietary decisions, to embrace a lifestyle that fosters sustained well-being, and to be agents of positive change on both societal and environmental fronts.

As we journey through the pages of this book, may the importance of healthy eating become not just a concept but a guiding principle—a principle that leads us toward a life characterized by vitality, balance, and a profound connection to the world of nutrition.

Chapter 2: The Fundamentals of Nutrition

In this second chapter, we embark on an enlightening journey into the essential building blocks of nutrition, unveiling the intricate web of macronutrients, micronutrients, and hydration that sustains our health and well-being.

Let's explore each of the three subchapters in greater depth, enriching our understanding of the vital role they play in our lives.

2.1 Macronutrients: Carbohydrates, Proteins, and Fats

Carbohydrates

Carbohydrates are one of the primary macronutrients that serve as the body's main source of energy. They encompass a diverse array of compounds, including sugars, starches, and dietary fiber. Carbohydrates can be found in an assortment of foods, from grains, fruits, and vegetables to dairy products.

They provide readily available energy, making them particularly crucial for activities requiring quick bursts of power, such as sprinting or mental tasks. Distinguishing between simple carbohydrates, like those found in candy, and complex carbohydrates abundant in whole grains and legumes empowers individuals to optimize energy intake and stabilize blood sugar levels.

Proteins

Proteins, often referred to as the "building blocks of life," hold an integral role in numerous bodily functions. They are composed of amino acids, which are essential for tissue growth, repair, and maintenance. Dietary sources of protein are rich and diverse, encompassing animal-based options like meat, fish, and eggs, as well as plant-based alternatives such as legumes, tofu, and nuts.

A balanced protein intake is vital for supporting muscle mass, immune system function, and the synthesis of enzymes and hormones.

Fats

Dietary fats represent another vital macronutrient, serving as an efficient energy reservoir, protecting vital organs, and facilitating the absorption of fat-soluble vitamins (A, D, E, and K). Fat sources can be categorized into saturated, monounsaturated, and polyunsaturated fats, each with its own impact on health.

For instance, avocados and olive oil are rich sources of heart-healthy monounsaturated fats, while saturated fats, primarily found in animal products and some processed foods, should be consumed in moderation. Moreover, an understanding of essential fatty acids, like omega-3 and omega-6, contributes to informed choices about dietary fat composition and its impact on cardiovascular health.

2.2 Micronutrients: Essential Vitamins and Minerals

Essential Vitamins

Vitamins are organic compounds that are indispensable for various biochemical processes within the body. These micronutrients are essential for maintaining health and preventing diseases.

For instance, vitamin C, found in citrus fruits and leafy greens, plays a pivotal role in immune function and collagen synthesis. Vitamin D, synthesized in the skin in response to sunlight, is critical for bone health.

Understanding the diverse roles of vitamins in promoting health and well-being empowers individuals to select a balanced diet rich in these vital compounds.

Essential Minerals

Minerals, inorganic nutrients, play a critical role in maintaining various physiological functions. Examples include calcium, vital for bone and teeth health, and iron, which is essential for oxygen transport in the blood.

The availability of minerals in foods varies, with sources ranging from dairy products to leafy greens and lean meats. A nuanced understanding of mineral intake, its absorption, and factors influencing mineral bioavailability assists in preventing deficiencies and ensuring optimal health.

2.3 Hydration and Water Consumption

Hydration transcends the boundaries of macronutrients and micronutrients, standing as a cornerstone of well-being. Water is essential for nearly every bodily function, from regulating body temperature to transporting nutrients and oxygen, removing waste products, and cushioning vital organs.

Understanding the significance of adequate hydration, as well as recognizing the subtle signs of dehydration, is paramount for maintaining health. Factors that influence individual hydration needs include age, physical activity level, climate, and overall health status.

For example, athletes and those in hot climates may require more fluids to compensate for increased sweat loss. Calculating daily fluid needs becomes imperative, and the "eight-by-eight" rule (eight 8-ounce glasses of water a day) provides a helpful baseline for most individuals.

Moreover, the impact of various beverages on hydration merits exploration. While water remains the gold standard for maintaining proper hydration, other beverages, such as herbal teas and natural fruit juices, can contribute to overall fluid intake.

However, some beverages, including sugary sodas and highly caffeinated drinks, may have diuretic effects and warrant moderation.

As we conclude this chapter, we have journeyed through the intricate world of macronutrients, micronutrients, and the vital role of hydration in nourishing our bodies.

Armed with this comprehensive knowledge, individuals are better equipped to make informed dietary choices that promote vitality, longevity, and sustained well-being throughout their lives.

Chapter 3: Benefits of Adopting a Real Food Diet

In this enlightening chapter, we embark on an exploration of the multifaceted advantages that come with embracing a real food diet—a nutritional approach that prioritizes unprocessed, nutrient-dense, and minimally refined foods.

As we delve deeper into the three subchapters, we will uncover the profound impact of such a diet on our health, vitality, and disease prevention.

3.1 Improved Digestive Health

A flourishing digestive system is the cornerstone of overall well-being, and adopting a real food diet can lead to substantial improvements:

Enhanced Gut Microbiota

Real foods, rich in dietary fiber, prebiotics, and essential nutrients, create a nurturing environment for beneficial gut bacteria. A diverse and balanced gut microbiome not only aids in efficient digestion but also plays a pivotal role in immune system regulation, metabolic processes, and even influences mental health.

Reduced Digestive Discomfort

One of the remarkable benefits of a real food diet is the avoidance of many additives, preservatives, and artificial ingredients commonly found in processed foods. This can lead to reduced digestive discomfort, such as bloating, gas, and indigestion, fostering a more pleasant and comfortable eating experience.

Digestive Disorders Prevention

A real food diet, characterized by its emphasis on whole, unprocessed ingredients, can reduce the risk of developing digestive disorders like irritable bowel syndrome (IBS) and diverticulitis. The avoidance of triggers such as excess sugar and highly processed foods is a key preventive measure.

Understanding the intricate interplay between diet and digestive health empowers individuals to make informed choices that not only enhance their comfort but also contribute to long-term well-being.

3.2 Increased Energy and Vitality

Sustained energy and vitality are the cornerstones of a fulfilling life, and a real food diet can significantly contribute to achieving these goals:

Balanced Blood Sugar

Real foods, especially those rich in complex carbohydrates like whole grains, legumes, and vegetables, promote stable blood sugar levels. This leads to sustained energy throughout the day, minimizing the energy spikes and crashes often associated with refined sugars and processed foods.

Nutrient-Rich Fuel

Nutrient-dense real foods provide the body with a consistent supply of essential vitamins, minerals, and antioxidants. These compounds are integral to cellular energy production and help combat oxidative stress, which can sap vitality.

Optimized Hydration

Proper hydration is paramount for maintaining energy levels. Real foods, particularly fruits and vegetables, are rich in water content, contributing to hydration. Even mild dehydration can lead to fatigue and reduced cognitive function.

By prioritizing a real food diet, individuals ensure they are providing their bodies with the necessary resources to maintain sustained energy and vitality throughout their daily activities.

3.3 Reduced Risk of Chronic Diseases

One of the most compelling benefits of adopting a real food diet is its potential to mitigate the risk of chronic diseases:

Heart Health

A diet anchored in real foods, particularly those rich in healthy fats like omega-3 fatty acids found in fatty fish, can significantly reduce the risk of heart disease. These fats lower levels of bad cholesterol (LDL) and triglycerides while promoting good cholesterol (HDL).

Weight Management

Real foods, due to their high fiber content and nutrient density, promote satiety, making it easier to achieve and maintain a healthy weight. Obesity, a significant risk factor for numerous chronic diseases, becomes less likely when real foods constitute the foundation of one's diet.

Diabetes Prevention

Stable blood sugar levels, a hallmark of a real food diet, reduce the risk of type 2 diabetes. Furthermore, a real food approach can be instrumental in managing blood sugar for individuals already diagnosed with diabetes.

Cancer Risk Reduction

A diet abundant in whole, unprocessed foods, particularly vegetables and fruits, is associated with a decreased risk of certain cancers. These foods are rich in antioxidants and phytochemicals that combat cell damage, inflammation, and the development of cancerous cells.

The benefits of adopting a real food diet extend far beyond enhanced digestion, increased energy, and reduced chronic disease risk.

This chapter underscores the transformative power of real food choices, motivating readers to embrace this path to well-being and longevity.

By nurturing a symbiotic relationship with food, individuals can harness the profound advantages of real food nutrition, thus enhancing their overall quality of life.

Chapter 4: Processed Foods vs. Real Foods

In this pivotal chapter, we embark on an enlightening journey into the essential dichotomy between processed foods and real foods. By delving deep into the intricate details and subtleties that distinguish these two dietary categories, we gain profound insights into the profound impact they have on our health, well-being, and the overall quality of our lives.

Let us embark on a comprehensive exploration of each of the three subchapters, unveiling the multifaceted nature of this crucial dietary distinction.

4.1 What Are Processed Foods

Understanding Processed Foods
Processed foods encompass a wide and diverse array of food products that have undergone varying degrees of alterations from their natural state.

These alterations can span the continuum from minimal processing techniques, such as freezing or drying, to extensive modifications involving the addition of artificial flavors, preservatives, sweeteners, and a multitude of chemical additives.

Processed foods can be found in various forms, including canned goods, packaged snacks, sugary beverages, and ready-made meals. Their primary attributes often prioritize convenience, extended shelf life, and flavor enhancement over intrinsic nutritional value.

Categorizing Processed Foods

To comprehensively grasp the world of processed foods, it's essential to systematically categorize them based on the extent of processing:

- **Minimally Processed Foods**
  This category includes foods that have undergone minimal alterations to enhance their shelf life or convenience. Examples include pre-washed and bagged salad greens, frozen vegetables, and pasteurized milk.

- **Moderately Processed Foods**
  Foods within this category undergo moderate processing and frequently include the addition of ingredients for flavor enhancement or preservation. Examples comprise canned soups, deli meats, and flavored yogurt.

- **Highly Processed Foods**
  These foods undergo extensive processing and typically contain a multitude of additives, preservatives, and refined ingredients. Highly processed foods are often found in fast-food items, sugary cereals, and most packaged snacks.

4.2 Issues with Processed Foods

The Pitfalls of Processed Foods

While processed foods undoubtedly offer convenience and a longer shelf life, they are fraught with several issues that can have adverse consequences on health and overall well-being:

Nutrient Depletion

The extensive processing that many foods undergo can strip them of essential nutrients, leaving them significantly less nutritious than their whole counterparts. This phenomenon is often referred to as "empty calories," where foods provide energy but little nutritional value.

Excessive Sugar, Salt, and Unhealthy Fats

Processed foods are often laden with excessive amounts of added sugars, sodium, and unhealthy trans fats. These elements contribute to various health issues, including obesity, heart disease, and hypertension.

Artificial Additives

Processed foods frequently feature artificial flavors, colors, and preservatives. These additives have raised concerns about potential health risks, including allergic reactions and potential adverse effects on children's behavior.

Lack of Dietary Fiber

Highly processed foods are typically low in dietary fiber, a critical component for digestive health and satiety. The absence of fiber can lead to digestive discomfort and overeating, as it fails to provide the feelings of fullness and satisfaction that whole foods offer.

Impact on Health

A diet that heavily relies on highly processed foods is associated with an elevated risk of obesity, diabetes, heart disease, and certain types of cancer. It can also lead to digestive issues, energy fluctuations, and an increased propensity for overconsumption due to reduced satiety.

Furthermore, the high sugar content in many processed foods can contribute to dental problems and chronic inflammation, which is linked to various diseases.

4.3 How to Identify Real Foods

Characteristics of Real Foods

Real foods, in stark contrast to their processed counterparts, are typically whole, unaltered, and brimming with nutrients. They offer numerous health benefits:

- **Unprocessed or Minimally Processed**
  Real foods are often found in their natural state or have undergone minimal processing. Examples encompass fresh fruits, vegetables, whole grains, lean proteins, and unprocessed dairy products.

- **Nutrient-Rich**
  They are naturally abundant in essential vitamins, minerals, antioxidants, and dietary fiber, all of which play pivotal roles in promoting overall health. These nutrients are not artificially added but are intrinsic to the food.

- **Simple Ingredient Lists**
  Real foods boast straightforward ingredient lists, with easily recognizable components. They are not laden with a multitude of additives or artificial substances. In essence, the ingredient list resembles what one might find in their own kitchen when preparing homemade meals.

- **Short Shelf Life**
  Owing to the absence of artificial preservatives, real foods tend to have a shorter shelf life. This underscores the significance of embracing freshness and seasonality in one's diet, as these foods are often more perishable.

- **Label Reading and Food Sourcing**
  To master the art of identifying real foods, it is imperative to educate oneself about reading food labels. This entails scrutinizing ingredient lists and being vigilant about recognizing additives,

preservatives, and hidden sugars. Additionally, sourcing food from local, sustainable producers can be instrumental in ensuring the authenticity and quality of the foods consumed.

By cultivating a profound understanding of the distinctions between processed and real foods, individuals can make conscious dietary decisions that prioritize their health, well-being, and longevity.

This chapter serves as a beacon of knowledge, shedding light on the pivotal role that food choices play in shaping our lives. It empowers readers to embark on a transformative journey towards a more nourishing, healthful, and sustainable diet that enriches their overall quality of life.

Chapter 5: Planning Healthy Meals

In this essential chapter, we embark on a journey of meal planning, a cornerstone of a nutritious and sustainable diet. By delving deep into the intricacies of planning healthy meals, we empower ourselves to make conscious, well-balanced food choices that promote vitality and well-being.

Let's explore each of the three subchapters in depth, unveiling the secrets to crafting nourishing and satisfying meals.

5.1 Creating a Meal Plan

The Art of Meal Planning

Meal planning is a strategic approach to structuring your daily and weekly meals. It involves carefully selecting foods and recipes to ensure a well-rounded, nutritious diet. Here's how to master the art of meal planning:

Set Clear Goals

Begin by establishing clear dietary goals, whether they're focused on weight management, health improvement, or specific nutritional needs (e.g., more fruits and vegetables, less sugar). Your goals will guide your meal planning choices.

Balanced Nutrition

Create meals that encompass a balance of macronutrients (carbohydrates, proteins, and fats) and micronutrients (vitamins and minerals). Aim for variety by incorporating foods from different food groups to maximize nutrient intake.

Grocery List

Based on your meal plan, create a comprehensive grocery list. Organizing your shopping list by food categories and sticking to it can help you make healthier choices at the store.

Preparation

Plan for meal preparation time by choosing recipes that fit your schedule. Consider batch cooking and meal prepping to save time and ensure you have healthy options readily available.

Flexibility

Allow for flexibility in your meal plan to accommodate unexpected events or changes in your schedule. Having a few quick and healthy go-to options can be a lifesaver on busy days.

5.2 Portion Control and Serving Sizes

Mastering Portion Control

Portion control is essential for managing calorie intake and preventing overeating. Here's how to master it:

- **Understand Serving Sizes**
  Familiarize yourself with standard serving sizes for different food groups. Tools like measuring cups and food scales can be useful for accurate portion control.

- **Mindful Eating**
  Practice mindful eating by paying attention to hunger and fullness cues. Eat slowly and savor each bite, which can help prevent overindulgence.

- **Plate Composition**
  Aim to fill half your plate with vegetables, one-quarter with lean protein, and one-quarter with whole grains. This balanced

plate composition promotes optimal
nutrition and satiety.

- **Avoid Distractions**
  Eating in front of the TV or computer can
  lead to mindless overeating. Focus on
  your meal and savor the flavors.

- **Use Smaller Plates**
  Using smaller plates and bowls can
  visually trick your brain into feeling
  satisfied with smaller portions.

5.3 Eating at Regular Intervals

The Importance of Regular Meals

Eating at regular intervals is crucial for
maintaining steady energy levels and preventing
overeating. Consider these principles:

- **Balanced Snacking**
  Include balanced snacks between meals to
  keep hunger at bay and maintain blood

sugar levels. Opt for whole foods like fruit, yogurt, or nuts.

- **Don't Skip Meals**
  Skipping meals can lead to excessive hunger, making it more likely to overindulge later in the day. Aim to have three balanced meals and, if necessary, healthy snacks.

- **Consistency**
  Try to eat meals and snacks at roughly the same times each day to establish a routine. This helps regulate your body's hunger and satiety signals.

- **Hydration**
  Don't forget to stay hydrated throughout the day. Sometimes thirst is mistaken for hunger.

- **Listen to Your Body**
  Pay attention to your body's hunger and fullness cues. Eat when you're hungry and stop when you're satisfied.

By mastering the art of meal planning, portion control, and eating at regular intervals, you'll be equipped to create a sustainable and nutritious eating pattern that supports your health and well-being.

This chapter provides the foundational knowledge and practical skills needed to make informed choices and develop lifelong healthy eating habits.

Chapter 6: Key Ingredients in a Real Food Diet

In this chapter, we embark on a culinary exploration of the fundamental components that constitute a real food diet. These key ingredients form the foundation of a wholesome and nourishing way of eating.

By diving deep into each of the three subchapters, we'll uncover the nuances of sourcing quality proteins, embracing complex carbohydrates and fiber, and selecting healthy fats and oils to create a balanced and health-enhancing diet.

6.1 Sourcing Quality Proteins

Understanding Quality Proteins

Proteins are the building blocks of life, and sourcing high-quality protein sources is a cornerstone of a real food diet. It involves selecting proteins that are minimally processed, ethically raised, and sustainably sourced. Examples of quality protein sources include:

- **Lean Meats**
  Choose lean cuts of meat from animals raised in humane and sustainable conditions. Grass-fed beef, pasture-raised poultry, and wild-caught fish are excellent options.

- **Plant-Based Proteins**
  For those following a vegetarian or vegan diet, plant-based protein sources such as legumes (lentils, chickpeas), tofu, tempeh, and quinoa offer ample protein content.

- **Dairy Products**
  If consuming dairy, opt for minimally processed and organic dairy products. Greek yogurt, cottage cheese, and high-quality cheeses can be part of a balanced real food diet.

- **Eggs**
  Eggs from pasture-raised chickens provide a rich source of protein and essential nutrients.

Benefits of Quality Proteins

Quality proteins not only provide essential amino acids for muscle repair and growth but also offer a range of essential nutrients, including vitamins, minerals, and healthy fats. Additionally, they are often free from antibiotics and hormones commonly found in conventionally raised animal products.

6.2 Complex Carbohydrates and Fiber

Embracing Complex Carbohydrates
Complex carbohydrates are an essential component of a real food diet, providing sustained energy and a wealth of nutrients. These carbohydrates are found in whole, unprocessed foods, such as:

- **Whole Grains**
  Whole grains like brown rice, quinoa, oats, and whole wheat pasta are rich sources of complex carbohydrates and fiber.

- **Vegetables**
  Non-starchy vegetables, such as leafy greens, broccoli, and bell peppers, are carbohydrate sources packed with vitamins, minerals, and fiber.

- **Legumes**
  Beans, lentils, and chickpeas are not only rich in complex carbohydrates but also provide plant-based protein and fiber.

The Role of Fiber

Fiber is a critical component of complex carbohydrates and plays a vital role in digestive health, blood sugar regulation, and satiety. A real food diet emphasizes high-fiber foods, which can help prevent constipation, reduce the risk of chronic diseases, and support weight management.

6.3 Healthy Fats and Oils

Selecting Healthy Fats

Healthy fats are an integral part of a real food diet and are essential for various bodily functions. When choosing fats and oils, focus on:

- **Monounsaturated Fats**
  Found in foods like avocados, olive oil, and nuts, monounsaturated fats are

associated with heart health and overall well-being.

- **Polyunsaturated Fats**
  Omega-3 and Omega-6 fatty acids, found in fatty fish (salmon, mackerel), flaxseeds, and walnuts, have anti-inflammatory properties and support brain health.

- **Coconut Oil**
  This saturated fat source has gained popularity for its potential health benefits, particularly in cooking and baking.

The Importance of Balance

A real food diet emphasizes the importance of a balanced intake of fats. While healthy fats offer numerous benefits, it's crucial to moderate saturated fats and avoid trans fats, which are often found in processed and fried foods.

By embracing quality proteins, complex carbohydrates, fiber-rich foods, and healthy fats and oils, individuals can craft a real food diet that nourishes their bodies, supports their health, and promotes overall well-being.

This chapter serves as a culinary guide, empowering readers to make informed choices that elevate their dietary habits and enhance their quality of life.

Chapter 7: Preparing and Cooking Healthy Meals

In this comprehensive exploration of Chapter 7, we embark on a culinary journey that delves into the art and science of preparing and cooking healthy meals, an essential component of a real food diet.

By mastering these skills, individuals can not only elevate the flavor and enjoyment of their meals but also make significant contributions to their overall well-being.

Let's delve deep into each of the three subchapters, uncovering the secrets of healthy cooking techniques, the importance of avoiding excess sugar and salt, and the significance of safe food storage.

7.1 Healthy Cooking Techniques

The Art of Healthy Cooking

Healthy cooking techniques are the backbone of preparing real food meals that are both delicious and nutritious. It's crucial to understand and master these techniques to ensure that the integrity of the ingredients is preserved. Here are some fundamental techniques:

- **Steaming**
  Steaming is a gentle cooking method that preserves the nutrients and natural flavors of vegetables. It involves cooking food over boiling water, allowing it to retain its freshness and vitality.

- **Baking and Roasting**
  Baking and roasting meats, poultry, and vegetables with minimal added fats can create delicious, crispy textures while preserving their nutritional value. These methods allow the natural sugars in foods to caramelize, enhancing their flavor.

- **Sautéing and Stir-Frying**
  Quick-cooking methods like sautéing and stir-frying require minimal oil and are perfect for locking in the flavors of vegetables, lean proteins, and whole grains. They result in dishes that are both flavorful and nutritious.

- **Grilling**
  Grilling is a fantastic way to add a smoky flavor to foods without excessive use of fats. It's particularly well-suited for lean meats, fish, and vegetables. The high heat of the grill can create beautiful charred textures.

Balancing Flavors

Healthy cooking techniques often prioritize the use of herbs, spices, and other flavor-enhancing ingredients to replace excessive salt and sugar. Fresh herbs like basil, cilantro, and rosemary, as well as aromatic ingredients like garlic, ginger, and citrus zest, can elevate dishes without relying on unhealthy additives.

By experimenting with a wide range of seasonings, individuals can discover exciting and healthy ways to enhance their meals.

7.2 Avoiding Excess Sugar and Salt

The Perils of Excess Sugar

Excessive sugar consumption is associated with a host of health problems, including obesity, type 2 diabetes, heart disease, and dental issues. In a real food diet, sweetness can be derived from natural sources such as fruits, honey, and maple syrup, reducing the need for added sugars.

Minimizing Salt Intake

High salt intake is linked to hypertension and an increased risk of heart disease. A real food approach often involves less salt, and instead, flavors are enhanced through the use of herbs, spices, and healthy fats. By using these flavor enhancers thoughtfully, individuals can reduce their reliance on salt while enjoying delicious meals.

The Importance of Label Reading

When purchasing packaged foods, it's essential to read labels carefully to identify hidden sugars and excessive sodium content. Opt for products with no added sugars or low sodium levels. Understanding food labels empowers consumers to make informed choices that align with their real food goals.

7.3 Safe Food Storage

Preserving Freshness and Safety

Safe food storage is paramount for maintaining the quality and safety of real foods. Here are some practical tips:

- **Refrigeration**
  Perishable items such as meats, dairy products, and fresh produce should be promptly refrigerated to prevent spoilage. Keeping the refrigerator at the appropriate temperature (usually 40°F or 4°C) is essential.

- **Freezing**
  Freezing is an effective way to extend the shelf life of foods while preserving their nutritional value. Proper packaging, such as airtight containers or freezer bags, is crucial to prevent freezer burn and maintain freshness.

- **Labeling**

  Labeling items in the freezer with the date of storage helps track freshness and reduce food waste. This practice ensures that foods are consumed before their quality deteriorates.

Safe Food Handling

Practicing proper food handling techniques is essential to prevent foodborne illnesses. This includes washing hands and utensils regularly, especially when handling raw meats, and avoiding cross-contamination.

By mastering healthy cooking techniques, avoiding excess sugar and salt, and practicing safe food storage, individuals can unlock the full potential of a real food diet. These culinary skills not only enhance the nutritional value of meals but also contribute to healthier, more enjoyable eating habits.

Chapter 8: Eating Out Healthily

In this chapter, we embark on a culinary adventure that takes us beyond the comforts of our home kitchen and into the world of dining out while maintaining a commitment to a real food diet. Whether you're at a restaurant or attending social events, you can make choices that align with your wholesome eating goals.

By delving deep into each of the three subchapters, we'll explore strategies for selecting restaurants with healthy options, gracefully navigating social events, and mastering the art of reading and understanding menus to make informed and satisfying choices.

8.1 Choosing Restaurants with Healthy Options

The Right Dining Destination

Selecting the right restaurant sets the tone for a successful healthy dining experience. Look for establishments that prioritize fresh, whole ingredients and offer options that align with real food principles:

- **Farm-to-Table Options**
  Seek out restaurants that emphasize farm-to-table dining. These establishments often source their ingredients locally and seasonally, ensuring freshness and quality.

- **Customizable Menus**
  Venues that allow you to customize your order are gems. They provide flexibility in choosing ingredients, such as opting for salad greens instead of fries as a side.

- **Health-Conscious Cuisine**
  Restaurants explicitly promoting health-conscious dining are more likely to offer real food options. Look for terms like "healthy," "light," or "wholesome" on menus.

Research Before You Dine

In the digital age, many restaurants offer their menus online, along with detailed nutritional information. Take advantage of this resource by researching restaurant choices ahead of time. It empowers you to make informed decisions that align with your dietary goals.

8.2 Strategies for Healthy Eating at Social Events

Mastering Social Event Dining

Social events often present challenges to maintaining a real food diet, but with the right strategies, you can navigate them successfully:

- **Communicate Your Preferences**
  Don't hesitate to communicate your dietary preferences or restrictions with the host or event planner. Many hosts are accommodating and can provide healthier options or modify dishes to suit your needs.

- **Eat a Balanced Meal Beforehand**
  If you anticipate limited real food options at an event, consider eating a small, balanced meal or snack beforehand. This curbs your appetite and reduces the temptation to overindulge in less healthy choices.

- **Bring Your Own Real Food**
  To ensure you have a nutritious option to enjoy, consider bringing a dish or snack that aligns with your dietary goals to share at the event. This proactive approach ensures you won't go hungry and may even inspire others to make healthier choices.

- **Practice Portion Control**

  Faced with a buffet of tempting but less healthy options, practice moderation. Take smaller portions of indulgent foods and fill the rest of your plate with healthier options, such as salads, lean proteins, and vegetables.

8.3 How to Read and Understand Menus

Decoding the Menu

Mastering the skill of reading and understanding menus is pivotal to making healthy choices when dining out:

- **Focus on Descriptions**

  Pay close attention to menu descriptions. Dishes described as "grilled," "roasted," or "steamed" are often healthier choices than those described as "fried" or "smothered."

- **Portion Size Awareness**
  Be mindful of portion sizes. Some restaurant servings can be larger than necessary. Consider sharing an entrée or ordering a half portion to avoid overeating.

- **Inquire About Ingredients**
  Don't hesitate to ask your server about specific ingredients or preparations. They can provide valuable information about how dishes are prepared and may be able to accommodate special requests based on your dietary preferences.

Utilizing Menu Categories

Many menus feature categories that can guide you in identifying real food options that align with your dietary preferences. Look for categories such as "vegetarian," "gluten-free," or "low-calorie" to help narrow down your choices.

By honing your skills in selecting restaurants with healthy options, gracefully navigating social events, and deciphering menus to make informed choices, you can confidently enjoy dining out while staying true to a real food diet.

This chapter empowers readers to savor the pleasures of restaurant dining and social gatherings without compromising their commitment to wholesome eating, ultimately enhancing their overall quality of life.

Chapter 9: Nutrition for Different Life Stages

In this comprehensive chapter, we embark on a profound exploration of the various life stages and how nutrition plays an instrumental role in shaping the health and well-being of individuals at each juncture.

From the delicate phases of pregnancy and breastfeeding, the formative years of childhood, to the graceful transition into older adulthood, nutrition is an ever-present and evolving factor that influences growth, development, and overall vitality.

Let's delve deeper into each of the three subchapters, gaining a richer understanding of the significance of nutrition during pregnancy and breastfeeding, child feeding and nutrition for kids, and the nuanced considerations in older adulthood.

9.1 Nutrition During Pregnancy and Breastfeeding

Nourishing Two Lives

Pregnancy and breastfeeding are profound life stages that usher in a cascade of physiological changes, demanding meticulous attention to nutrition. It's a time when the nutritional choices of a mother directly impact her health and the healthy development of her baby. Key considerations include:

- **Folic Acid and Prenatal Vitamins**
  Adequate folic acid intake is critical during pregnancy as it helps prevent neural tube defects. Prenatal vitamins may be recommended to ensure essential nutrient levels are met.

- **Balanced Diet**
  Pregnant and breastfeeding women require additional nutrients, including protein, calcium, iron, and omega-3 fatty acids. A balanced diet rich in fruits, vegetables, lean proteins, and whole grains is essential to provide the necessary building blocks for the developing baby.

- **Hydration**
  Staying well-hydrated is vital during pregnancy and breastfeeding. Proper hydration supports the increased fluid needs of both the mother and the baby.

Nutrient-Dense Choices

During pregnancy and breastfeeding, it's imperative to focus on nutrient-dense foods that provide essential vitamins, minerals, and antioxidants.

These foods not only support the growth and development of the baby but also contribute to the overall health and well-being of the mother.

9.2 Child Feeding and Nutrition for Kids

Building Healthy Foundations

Childhood represents a crucial phase for establishing lifelong eating habits and ensuring optimal growth and development. Nutritional considerations for kids include:

- **Balanced Meals**
  Children benefit from balanced meals that encompass a variety of foods from all food groups. This approach not only supports

growth but also helps prevent nutrient deficiencies.

- **Healthy Snacking**
  Encouraging nutritious snacks like fruits, vegetables, yogurt, and nuts not only helps children meet their nutritional needs but also instills healthy eating habits from an early age.

- **Avoiding Excess Sugar**
  Limiting sugar intake is essential for preventing dental issues, maintaining a healthy weight, and promoting overall health. Encouraging whole foods over sugary snacks and beverages fosters better dietary choices.

Positive Food Experiences

Creating positive food experiences for children can have a lasting impact on their relationship with food. It involves exposing them to a variety of flavors and textures, involving them in meal preparation, and fostering a positive mealtime environment.

9.3 Nutrition in Older Adulthood

Aging Gracefully

As individuals transition into older adulthood, their nutritional needs evolve, presenting unique challenges and opportunities for maintaining health and vitality. Key considerations include:

- **Protein Intake**
  Older adults often require more protein to counteract age-related muscle loss and support bone health. Including lean meats, fish, legumes, and dairy products can help meet protein needs.

- **Calcium and Vitamin D**
  Adequate calcium and vitamin D intake are essential for preserving bone health and reducing the risk of fractures. Dairy

products, leafy greens, and fortified foods
are good sources.

- **Hydration**
  Staying adequately hydrated becomes
  increasingly important as people age.
  Dehydration can lead to a range of health
  issues, so seniors should prioritize water
  intake.

Maintaining Independence

Nutrition plays a significant role in preserving
independence and quality of life in older
adulthood. Adequate nutrient intake supports
cognitive function, immune health, and overall
vitality, allowing older adults to maintain an
active and independent lifestyle.

By comprehending the unique nutritional needs
and challenges posed by different life stages,
individuals can make informed dietary choices
that foster optimal health and well-being.

This chapter serves as a comprehensive guide, illuminating the complex interplay between nutrition and the various phases of life, ultimately enhancing the overall quality of life at each stage.

Chapter 10: Myths and Misconceptions in Nutrition

In this enlightening chapter, we embark on a journey through the often-confusing landscape of nutrition myths and misconceptions. Nutrition is a field rife with misinformation, and understanding the truth is pivotal to making informed dietary choices.

By delving into each of the three subchapters, we'll explore the process of debunking common myths, unravel the pitfalls of popular diets, and underscore the importance of nutrition education.

10.1 Debunking Common Myths

Separating Fact from Fiction

Nutrition myths have a remarkable ability to persist, often leading individuals down dietary paths that may not be rooted in scientific evidence. In this subchapter, we'll explore the process of debunking common myths, such as:

Myth 1: Carbohydrates are the Enemy

One prevalent myth suggests that carbohydrates are the root cause of weight gain and should be avoided at all costs. While it's true that excessive consumption of refined carbohydrates can lead to health issues, not all carbs are created equal.

Whole grains, fruits, and vegetables provide essential nutrients and fiber, promoting fullness and overall health. The key is to focus on complex carbohydrates and minimize simple sugars and refined grains.

Myth 2: Fat-Free is the Healthiest Option

The fat-free craze of the past led many to believe that eliminating all fats from their diets was the path to optimal health. However, fats are crucial for various bodily functions, including the absorption of fat-soluble vitamins and the maintenance of healthy cell membranes.

It's essential to differentiate between healthy fats (e.g., those found in avocados, nuts, and olive oil) and trans fats or excessive saturated fats, which can be harmful.

Myth 3: All Calories are Equal

The "calories in, calories out" concept suggests that weight management is solely about calorie balance. While calorie intake matters, the source of those calories is equally important.

Nutrient-dense foods provide more than just energy; they supply essential vitamins, minerals, and antioxidants crucial for overall health. A diet primarily composed of empty-calorie foods lacks these vital nutrients.

Myth 4: Supplements Can Replace Real Food

Supplements have their place, but they should not be seen as a substitute for a well-balanced diet. Real foods offer a symphony of nutrients, fiber, and phytonutrients that work together to support health. While supplements can address specific deficiencies, they cannot replicate the complexity of real foods.

Myth 5: Eating Healthy is Expensive

This myth often deters individuals from adopting a healthier diet. While some healthy foods can be costly, a well-planned real food diet doesn't have to break the bank. Seasonal, locally sourced produce, bulk grains, and smart meal planning can make nutritious eating affordable and accessible.

By dispelling these common myths, we pave the way for a more informed and balanced approach to nutrition. The key lies in embracing real fooding, making mindful choices, and understanding that a healthy diet is one that is both enjoyable and sustainable.

Empowering Through Knowledge

Debunking nutrition myths is a powerful tool for empowering individuals to make choices that align with their health goals. Understanding the scientific evidence behind dietary recommendations helps individuals navigate the sea of conflicting information.

10.2 Pitfalls of Popular Diets

The Promise and Peril of Diets

The world of dieting is a dynamic landscape, filled with trendy diets promising quick fixes and dramatic transformations. In this subchapter, we'll delve into the pitfalls of popular diets, including:

- **Fad Diets**
  Explore the allure and dangers of fad diets, from extreme low-carb diets to detox cleanses, and understand why they often fall short of delivering lasting results.

- **Restrictive Eating**
  Investigate the potential harms of overly restrictive eating patterns, such as those seen in very low-calorie diets and elimination diets.

- **Yo-Yo Dieting**
  Uncover the physical and psychological effects of yo-yo dieting, a cycle of weight loss and regain that can be detrimental to long-term health.

Promoting Sustainable Health

Recognizing the limitations and risks associated with popular diets is essential for fostering a sustainable approach to health. We'll explore the principles of balanced and evidence-based eating that can lead to lasting well-being.

10.3 The Importance of Nutrition Education

Equipping for Nutritional Literacy
Nutrition education is a powerful tool for equipping individuals with the knowledge and skills needed to make informed dietary choices. In this subchapter, we'll underscore the importance of nutrition education by:

- **Promoting Critical Thinking**
  Encourage critical thinking about dietary information and sources, enabling individuals to discern credible nutrition advice from sensationalized claims.

- **Lifelong Learning**
  Emphasize the value of ongoing nutrition education, as scientific understanding of nutrition evolves. Lifelong learners are

better equipped to adapt to new findings and make informed choices.

- **Community and School-Based Programs**
  Highlight the role of community and school-based nutrition programs in promoting nutritional literacy, especially among children and adolescents.

Nutrition as Empowerment

Nutrition education empowers individuals to take control of their health by making choices that align with their unique needs and goals. It also fosters a deeper appreciation for the vital role nutrition plays in overall well-being.

By delving into the world of nutrition myths, the pitfalls of popular diets, and the importance of nutrition education, this chapter equips readers with the tools needed to navigate the complex and often contradictory realm of dietary information.

It fosters a greater understanding of the science of nutrition, empowering individuals to make informed choices that enhance their health and quality of life.

Chapter 11: The Role of Nutrients in Health

In this enlightening chapter, we dive deep into the fundamental building blocks of nutrition and explore the pivotal role that nutrients play in shaping our health and well-being. Nutrients are the essential components of our diet, providing the raw materials needed for growth, energy, and the intricate biochemical processes that keep our bodies functioning optimally.

By delving into each of the three subchapters, we'll unravel the intricacies of essential nutrients, delve into the world of micronutrients (vitamins and minerals), and gain a comprehensive understanding of macronutrients (carbohydrates, proteins, and fats).

11.1 Exploring Essential Nutrients

The Nutritional Essentials

Essential nutrients are the cornerstone of a balanced and nourishing diet. They are classified into two main categories: macronutrients and micronutrients. Essential nutrients include:

- **Water**
  Often overlooked as a nutrient, water is indispensable for life. It plays a role in virtually every bodily function, from digestion and circulation to temperature regulation.

- **Macronutrients**
  These are nutrients required in larger quantities and include carbohydrates, proteins, and fats. They serve as the primary sources of energy and are essential for growth and repair.

- **Micronutrients**

  Micronutrients are required in smaller amounts but are no less critical. They encompass vitamins and minerals, which act as cofactors in countless biochemical reactions and are essential for overall health.

The Role of Essential Nutrients

Each essential nutrient plays a specific role in maintaining health and well-being. For example, carbohydrates provide quick energy, proteins are the building blocks of tissues, and fats are crucial for cell structure.

Understanding the roles of these nutrients empowers individuals to make dietary choices that align with their unique needs and goals.

11.2 Micronutrients: Vitamins and Minerals

Vitamins: Nature's Multitaskers

Vitamins are organic compounds that play vital roles in various physiological processes. They are classified into two groups:

- **Fat-Soluble Vitamins**
  This group includes vitamins A, D, E, and K, which dissolve in fat and are stored in the body. They play roles in vision, bone health, antioxidant protection, and blood clotting, among others.

- **Water-Soluble Vitamins**
  Water-soluble vitamins, such as vitamin C and the B-complex vitamins, are not stored in the body to the same extent as fat-soluble vitamins. They play essential roles in energy metabolism, immune function, and skin health, among other functions.

Minerals: The Body's Building Blocks

Minerals are inorganic nutrients that serve as structural components, electrolytes, and cofactors for various biochemical reactions. Key minerals include:

- **Calcium**
  Critical for bone and teeth health, muscle function, and blood clotting.

- **Iron**
  Essential for oxygen transport in the blood and overall energy metabolism.

- **Sodium and Potassium**
  Electrolytes that help maintain fluid balance and nerve function.

- **Magnesium**
  Involved in muscle and nerve function, blood glucose control, and bone health.

The Micronutrient Puzzle

Micronutrients work in concert to support health and well-being. A deficiency or excess of any one micronutrient can disrupt this delicate balance and lead to health issues.

Understanding how to obtain a wide variety of vitamins and minerals from a balanced diet is key to maintaining optimal health.

11.3 Understanding Macronutrients: Carbohydrates, Proteins, and Fats

Macronutrients in Depth

Macronutrients are the nutritional powerhouses that provide energy and the structural elements needed for growth and repair. Let's explore each macronutrient category in detail:

- **Carbohydrates**
  Carbohydrates are the body's primary source of energy. They can be classified into simple and complex carbs, with complex carbs providing sustained energy and fiber for digestive health.

- **Proteins**
  Proteins are the building blocks of life, composed of amino acids. They play roles in tissue repair, immune function, enzyme production, and more. Understanding protein quality and sources empowers individuals to meet their protein needs.

- **Fats**
  Fats are often misunderstood, but they are essential for health. They provide long-term energy storage, cushion organs, and are integral to cell membranes. Distinguishing between healthy fats (unsaturated fats) and unhealthy fats (saturated and trans fats) is crucial for

making dietary choices that support heart health.

Balancing Macronutrients

A balanced diet includes an appropriate mix of carbohydrates, proteins, and fats. Understanding one's energy needs, activity level, and individual dietary preferences is vital for achieving this balance.

By gaining a comprehensive understanding of essential nutrients, exploring the world of micronutrients (vitamins and minerals), and delving into the roles of macronutrients (carbohydrates, proteins, and fats), readers can unlock the key to optimal nutrition.

This chapter serves as a foundational guide, illuminating the intricate web of nutrients that sustain life and well-being, ultimately empowering individuals to make informed dietary choices that enhance their overall quality of life.

Chapter 12: Superfoods and Functional Foods

In this captivating chapter, we delve into the world of superfoods and functional foods, exploring the exceptional nutritional qualities that make these foods stand out.

Superfoods are nutrient-packed powerhouses known for their exceptional health benefits, while functional foods are everyday edibles with specific health-enhancing properties.

By delving into each of the three subchapters, we'll unravel the mysteries of superfoods, uncover the potential of functional foods for optimal health, and learn how to seamlessly incorporate these nutritional heroes into our daily diets.

12.1 What Are Superfoods?

The Nutritional Titans

Superfoods are not merely foods; they are exceptional nutrient powerhouses, lauded for their remarkable health benefits and unparalleled nutritional richness. This subchapter offers an in-depth exploration of these dietary marvels, beginning with:

- **Superfood Categories**
  Dive into the world of superfoods by uncovering the various categories they belong to. From the vibrant and antioxidant-rich berries, such as blueberries and acai, to the verdant and

nutrient-dense leafy greens like kale and spinach, superfoods offer a diverse array of choices.

- **Nutrient-Rich Profile**
  Delve deep into the nutrient profiles that set superfoods apart. These foods are brimming with essential vitamins, minerals, fiber, and antioxidants. Understanding the nutritional treasure trove they offer empowers you to make informed dietary choices.

- **Health Benefits**
  Explore the scientific evidence supporting the numerous health benefits linked to superfoods. From bolstering cognitive function and heart health to combating inflammation, these foods have earned their superlative status through rigorous research and a wealth of positive outcomes.

Superfoods in Context

While the allure of superfoods is undeniable, their true potential is realized when they become an integral part of a well-balanced diet.

This subchapter provides practical insights on how to incorporate these nutritional gems seamlessly into your daily culinary repertoire.

12.2 Functional Foods for Optimal Health

Everyday Heroes

Functional foods are the unsung heroes of our daily diet, offering tailored health benefits that go beyond basic nourishment. This subchapter uncovers the wide-ranging world of functional foods, including:

- **Examples of Functional Foods**
  Journey through a diverse array of functional foods commonly found in everyday meals. Explore the probiotic

richness of yogurt, the fiber-packed goodness of oats, and the omega-3 fatty acid bounty of salmon. These heroes of the kitchen offer unique health advantages.

- **Specific Health Benefits**
  Delve into the distinct health benefits associated with various functional foods. Witness how they can improve digestive health, support heart health by lowering cholesterol levels, enhance blood sugar control, and contribute to your overall well-being.

- **Bioactive Compounds**
  Gain a deeper understanding of the bioactive compounds present in functional foods. Discover how prebiotics, probiotics, dietary fiber, and a plethora of phytochemicals are the driving forces behind the health-boosting potential of these everyday edibles.

Functional Foods as Preventive Medicine

Functional foods are not just delicious additions to your diet; they serve as powerful tools for proactive health maintenance. Explore how incorporating these foods can be a transformative step on your journey toward optimal well-being.

12.3 Incorporating Superfoods into Your Diet

Practical Guidance

Making superfoods a regular part of your diet need not be complex. This subchapter provides pragmatic guidance on:

- **Selecting Superfoods**
  Learn the art of choosing, storing, and preparing superfoods to preserve their nutritional potency and vibrant flavors.

- **Incorporation Strategies**
  Discover creative and accessible methods for seamlessly integrating superfoods into your daily meals. Whether you're crafting vibrant and nutrient-packed smoothies, assembling superfood-infused salads, concocting satisfying snacks, or preparing delectable main dishes, the culinary possibilities are endless.

- **Balanced Nutrition**
  Embrace the importance of incorporating superfoods within the context of a well-balanced diet. This ensures you receive a diverse spectrum of nutrients to support your holistic well-being.

Superfoods for the Long Haul

Sustainable and enjoyable consumption of superfoods is the key to reaping their enduring benefits. Explore how to make these foods a delightful and lasting part of your culinary journey, ensuring that their nutritional brilliance becomes a lifelong dietary companion.

By unraveling the mystique of superfoods, navigating the multifaceted world of functional foods, and offering practical strategies for seamlessly incorporating these nutritional powerhouses into your daily diet, this chapter equips you with the knowledge and tools to make informed dietary choices that elevate your overall well-being.

It invites you to embrace the culinary universe of foods that not only nourish your body but also foster enduring health and vitality for years to come.

Chapter 13: Nutrition for Athletic Performance

In this dynamic and comprehensive chapter, we embark on a journey into the realm of nutrition for athletic performance, uncovering the strategies and principles that enable athletes to reach the pinnacle of their abilities in sports and exercise.

Nutrition stands as one of the cornerstones of athletic success, and within this chapter, we delve deep into the art and science of optimally fueling your body for sports and exercise, navigating the intricate landscape of recovery nutrition and hydration, and gaining a nuanced understanding of the role of supplements in enhancing athletic prowess.

13.1 Fueling Your Body for Sports and Exercise

The Energy Equation

Athletic success hinges on the foundation of proper nutrition, which serves as the engine propelling performance. In this subchapter, we delve into the critical components of fueling your body for sports and exercise:

- **Energy Needs**
  Grasp the unique energy demands associated with various sports and exercises. Whether you're an endurance athlete, strength trainer, or engage in high-intensity interval training, recognizing the specific fueling requirements of your chosen activity is

paramount to achieving peak performance.

- **Macronutrient Balance**
  Gain a profound understanding of the ideal balance of carbohydrates, proteins, and fats tailored to athletic endeavors. Each macronutrient plays a distinct role in energy production, muscle repair, and overall stamina, and achieving the right equilibrium is key.

- **Timing and Pre-Workout Nutrition**
  Explore the science of meal timing and pre-workout nutrition. Learn how to optimize your meals to provide sustained energy, enhance endurance during exercise, and prime your body for the challenges ahead.

Performance Enhancement

Properly fueling your body before and during physical activity is the linchpin of achieving peak performance. Unlock the strategies and nutrition plans that can provide you with the competitive edge you seek, whether you're aiming for a personal best or vying for victory.

13.2 Recovery Nutrition and Hydration

The Vital Role of Recovery

Recovery nutrition is often the unsung hero of athletic performance. In this subchapter, we delve into the intricacies of post-exercise nutrition and hydration:

- **Nutrient Timing**
  Explore the significance of nutrient timing in the post-exercise phase. Properly timed meals and snacks are instrumental in facilitating muscle repair, replenishing glycogen stores, and minimizing the risk of injury.

- **Hydration**
  Understand the paramount importance of maintaining proper hydration levels

before, during, and after exercise. Dehydration can have a catastrophic impact on performance, hinder recovery, and even pose health risks.

- **Recovery Foods**
  Delve into the selection of recovery foods that support optimal recuperation. Nutrient-dense options rich in protein, carbohydrates, antioxidants, and anti-inflammatory compounds play a pivotal role in accelerating recovery and reducing post-exercise soreness.

Optimizing Recovery

An effective recovery plan can be a game-changer for athletes seeking peak performance. Learn how to tailor your post-exercise nutrition and hydration to enhance muscle repair, reduce muscle soreness, and set the stage for future athletic success.

13.3 Supplements for Athletes

Enhancing Performance Safely

Supplements have become an integral part of modern athletic nutrition, but navigating this landscape requires careful consideration. In this subchapter, we delve into the complex world of supplements for athletes:

- **Supplement Categories**
  Explore the diverse categories of supplements commonly used by athletes, including protein supplements, energy gels, electrolyte tablets, and performance-enhancing substances. Understand their specific roles and potential benefits.

- **Evaluating Supplement Safety**
  Grasp the critical importance of evaluating supplement safety and efficacy. Not all supplements are created equal, and making informed choices is essential to avoid potential health risks.

- **Regulations and Doping**
  Learn about the regulations and anti-doping rules governing supplements in competitive sports. Adherence to these regulations is crucial for preserving your athletic reputation, eligibility, and long-term health.

Supplements as Tools, Not Shortcuts

While supplements can be valuable tools in the athlete's arsenal, they should complement rather than replace a well-balanced diet. Discover how to use supplements judiciously and responsibly to enhance your nutrition plan, boost performance, and safeguard your health.

By immersing yourself in the strategies for fueling your body for sports and exercise, mastering the nuances of recovery nutrition and hydration, and gaining a comprehensive understanding of the role of supplements in enhancing athletic performance, this chapter equips you with the knowledge, insights, and practical guidance to optimize your nutritional approach as an athlete.

It invites you to embrace nutrition as a dynamic and integral component of your training regimen, unlocking your full potential for success in sports and physical activities.

Chapter 14: Nutrition and Mental Health

In this enlightening and pivotal chapter, we embark on a journey through the intricate relationship between nutrition and mental health, shedding light on how the foods we consume can significantly impact our psychological well-being.

The link between what we eat and our mental health is a burgeoning field of research, and within this chapter, we explore the profound concept of the gut-brain connection, uncover foods that support mental well-being, and delve into nutritional strategies for managing stress and anxiety.

14.1 The Gut-Brain Connection

The Enteric Nervous System

The gut-brain connection is a burgeoning field of research that reveals the intricate relationship between the digestive system and mental health. Within your gut lies the enteric nervous system, often referred to as the "second brain." This complex network of neurons is capable of independent decision-making and communicates extensively with your central nervous system. Here's a deeper dive:

- **The Enteric Nervous System**
  Your gut is home to an astounding number of neurons - approximately 100 million, which is more than in the spinal cord. These neurons allow your digestive system to function independently, controlling essential processes like peristalsis and enzyme secretion.

- **Microbiota and Mental Health**
  The gut microbiota, the diverse community of microorganisms residing in your intestines, plays a pivotal role in your mental health. Emerging research suggests that the composition of your gut bacteria can influence your mood, cognition, and susceptibility to conditions like depression and anxiety. A balanced gut microbiome is associated with better mental well-being.

- **Nutrition and Gut Health**
  Nutrition plays a vital role in maintaining a healthy gut and nurturing the gut-brain axis. Consuming a diet rich in fiber, fermented foods, and prebiotics can promote the growth of beneficial gut bacteria. These microbes produce neurotransmitters like serotonin, often dubbed the "feel-good" neurotransmitter, which can positively affect mood.

Healing the Gut-Brain Axis

Your dietary choices can significantly impact the health of your gut-brain axis. A diet that includes fiber-rich foods like whole grains and vegetables, fermented foods like yogurt and kimchi, and prebiotics like garlic and onions can foster a balanced and resilient gut microbiome. By nurturing your gut, you support not only your digestive health but also your mental well-being.

14.2 Foods That Support Mental Well-being

Nutritional Psychiatry

The emerging field of nutritional psychiatry underscores the profound link between diet and mental health. Your food choices can indeed influence your emotional well-being. Here's a closer look:

- **Mood-Boosting Foods**
  Certain foods have earned their reputation as mood enhancers. For

instance, fatty fish like salmon and mackerel are rich in omega-3 fatty acids, which have been linked to lower rates of depression. Berries, with their high antioxidant content, can protect brain cells from oxidative stress. Dark chocolate, in moderation, can stimulate the release of endorphins, promoting a sense of pleasure and relaxation.

- **Balanced Nutrition**
  The foundation of good mental health lies in balanced nutrition. A diet that includes whole grains, lean proteins like poultry and tofu, healthy fats like avocados and nuts, and a colorful array of fruits and vegetables provides essential nutrients for cognitive function and emotional stability. These nutrients include B vitamins, magnesium, and antioxidants.

- **Mindful Eating**
  Mindful eating is a practice that encourages you to savor each bite,

fostering a deeper connection between your food and your emotions. By eating mindfully, you become more attuned to your body's hunger and fullness cues, potentially preventing overeating and promoting a healthier relationship with food.

Fueling Your Mind

Your dietary choices are a potent tool for supporting mental well-being. By incorporating mood-boosting foods, maintaining a balanced diet rich in essential nutrients, and practicing mindful eating, you can take proactive steps toward cultivating a positive mindset and emotional resilience.

14.3 Nutritional Strategies for Stress and Anxiety

Managing the Anxieties of Life

Stress and anxiety are pervasive aspects of modern life, but your diet can play a significant role in managing these emotional challenges. Here are valuable strategies:

- **Adaptogenic Foods**
  Adaptogens are a class of herbs and foods that help the body adapt to stress. For example, ashwagandha, an adaptogenic herb, has been shown to reduce stress and anxiety by modulating the body's stress response. Dark chocolate, with its antioxidant properties and ability to promote relaxation, can be a soothing treat.

- **Relaxation-Inducing Nutrients**
  Certain nutrients have relaxation-inducing properties. Magnesium, found in foods like nuts and leafy greens, can relax muscles and reduce tension. B vitamins, particularly B6 and B12, are essential for neurotransmitter production and can play a role in mood regulation. Herbal teas like chamomile have a calming effect and can reduce anxiety symptoms.

- **Balancing Blood Sugar**

  Blood sugar fluctuations can contribute to mood swings and exacerbate anxiety. Consuming balanced meals and snacks that include complex carbohydrates, lean proteins, and healthy fats can help stabilize blood sugar levels. Avoiding excessive sugar and refined carbohydrates can prevent energy crashes and mood disturbances.

Empowering Your Emotional Resilience

Your diet can be a powerful ally in managing stress and anxiety effectively. By incorporating adaptogenic foods, prioritizing relaxation-inducing nutrients, and maintaining stable blood sugar levels through balanced nutrition, you can enhance your emotional resilience and reduce the impact of stress on your mental health.

This chapter invites you to explore the profound connection between nutrition and mental health, empowering you to make informed dietary choices that not only nourish your body but also foster emotional well-being and resilience. It underscores the notion that food is not merely fuel; it is a tool for nurturing a positive mindset and supporting mental wellness.

Chapter 15: Real Food for a Sustainable Future

In this final chapter, we shift our focus to the intersection of nutrition and sustainability, exploring how our dietary choices profoundly impact the health of our planet.

As global environmental challenges intensify, understanding the importance of sustainable food choices, reducing food waste, and mitigating the environmental impact of our diets becomes paramount for a sustainable future.

15.1 Sustainable Food Choices

The Nexus of Nutrition and Sustainability

The choices we make at the grocery store and in our kitchens have far-reaching implications for the environment. In this subchapter, we explore the concept of sustainable food choices:

- **Defining Sustainability** Sustainability in food is about the responsible use of resources to meet our dietary needs while considering the long-term health of ecosystems and communities. It encompasses not only environmental considerations but also social and economic factors. Sustainable food choices aim to strike a balance between these pillars.

- **Local and Seasonal Eating**
  One key sustainable practice is opting for local and seasonal foods. This approach reduces the carbon footprint associated with food transportation. By choosing produce and products grown or harvested nearby, consumers support local economies, reduce emissions from transport, and promote the resilience of local food systems.

- **Plant-Based Diets**
  Plant-based diets are increasingly recognized for their environmental advantages. Reducing meat consumption and incorporating more plant foods can significantly reduce greenhouse gas emissions and alleviate pressure on land and water resources. Plant-centric diets are not only nutritious but also contribute to sustainability by conserving resources and lowering the environmental burden of food production.

Eating for the Planet

Sustainable food choices empower individuals to be stewards of the Earth. By embracing practices such as local and seasonal eating and exploring plant-based diets, consumers can make conscious decisions that reduce their ecological footprint and support a healthier planet for future generations.

15.2 Reducing Food Waste

The Silent Sustainability Crisis

Food waste is a global issue that exacerbates hunger, strains environmental resources, and has economic repercussions. In this subchapter, we delve into the critical topic of reducing food waste:

- **Understanding Food Waste**
  Food waste occurs at various stages of the supply chain, from the farm to the consumer's table. It results from factors such as overproduction, inefficient

harvesting, cosmetic standards, and consumer behaviors. Recognizing the scope and causes of food waste is essential to addressing this complex issue.

- **Practical Strategies**
  Reducing food waste starts with practical strategies that individuals can adopt in their daily lives. Meal planning, proper food storage, and creative approaches to using leftovers are effective ways to minimize waste. Additionally, understanding expiration dates and learning to distinguish between "sell by" and "use by" labels can prevent unnecessary discarding of perfectly good food.

- **Community Initiatives**
  Beyond individual efforts, there are community-based initiatives and organizations dedicated to reducing food waste. Food rescue programs, food banks, and gleaning initiatives collect surplus

food and distribute it to those in need. These efforts not only combat food waste but also contribute to food security and support vulnerable populations.

The Power of Waste Reduction

Reducing food waste is a powerful strategy for promoting sustainability and combating hunger. By adopting mindful food practices at home and supporting organizations working toward food waste reduction, individuals can make a tangible and positive impact on both their communities and the environment.

15.3 The Environmental Impact of Diet Choices

Eating Green

Our dietary choices have a profound impact on the environment, influencing factors such as land and water use, greenhouse gas emissions, and the health of ecosystems. In this subchapter, we delve into the environmental implications of diet choices:

- **Water and Land Use**
  Different foods have varying water and land requirements for production. Livestock farming, particularly for beef, places substantial pressure on resources. Plant-based diets are generally more resource-efficient, requiring less land and water. Choosing foods with a lower environmental footprint can contribute to resource conservation.

- **Greenhouse Gas Emissions**
  The production and transportation of food are significant contributors to greenhouse gas emissions. Diets high in animal products, especially red meat, tend to have a larger carbon footprint. Shifting toward plant-centric diets and reducing meat consumption can help mitigate climate change by reducing emissions.

- **Sustainable Seafood**
  Seafood is a critical protein source for many, but overfishing and destructive fishing practices harm marine ecosystems. Sustainable seafood choices, guided by certifications like the Marine Stewardship Council (MSC) label, support responsible fishing practices that preserve ocean health and maintain fish populations.

A Path to Environmental Stewardship

Dietary choices are a potent lever for environmental change. By embracing sustainable food choices, reducing food waste, and understanding the environmental impact of their diets, individuals can become advocates for a more sustainable future.

These choices demonstrate that food is not merely nourishment but also a means of fostering a healthier planet for current and future generations.

By exploring the profound connection between nutrition and sustainability, individuals can make informed dietary choices that not only support personal health but also contribute to the well-being of the planet.

This chapter emphasizes the transformative power of food choices in addressing pressing environmental challenges and encourages readers to become active participants in building a more sustainable and prosperous future for all.

Conclusions

In this journey through the realms of nutrition and real fooding, we've embarked on a path to rediscover the profound impact that our dietary choices have on our health, our well-being, and our planet. As we conclude this book, let's reflect on some key takeaways:

1. **The Power of Real Food**
   Real food, unprocessed and close to its natural state, is a potent source of nourishment. It provides us with the essential nutrients our bodies need to thrive, and its simplicity is a testament to its wisdom.

2. **Nutrition is Personal**
   There is no one-size-fits-all approach to nutrition. Each of us is unique, and our dietary choices should reflect our individual needs, preferences, and health goals.

3. **Sustainability Matters**
   The foods we choose not only impact our personal health but also the health of our planet. Sustainable food choices can help mitigate environmental challenges and

create a brighter future for generations to come.

4. **The Journey Never Ends**
Our understanding of nutrition is continually evolving. Staying informed and open to new insights is an essential part of our ongoing journey toward healthier and more conscious eating.

5. **Action Transforms**
The knowledge gained from this book becomes truly powerful when put into action. Small, consistent changes in our food choices and habits can lead to profound transformations in our health and our lives.

As you close this book and embark on your own journey toward a healthier and more sustainable way of eating, remember that you hold the key to your own well-being.

I hope the information shared here serves as a guide and an inspiration as you navigate the world of nutrition and embrace the beauty of real food.

Thank you for joining me on this exploration, and may your path be filled with vitality, joy, and the simple pleasures of real, wholesome food.

For Further Information

If you'd like to delve deeper into nutrition, real fooding, and maintaining a healthy lifestyle, we recommend exploring the following resources:

Recommended Books

- Nutrition and You by Joan Salge Blake
- Real Food for a Balanced Life by Emily White
- In Defense of Food: An Eater's Manifesto by Michael Pollan
- The Omnivore's Dilemma: A Natural History of Four Meals by Michael Pollan

Websites and Blogs

- Academy of Nutrition and Dietetics (https://www.eatright.org/): Nutrition and healthy eating resources backed by registered dietitians.
- Real Food Dietitians(https://therealfoodrds.com/): Recipes and tips for a real food-based diet.
- Nutrition.gov (https://www.nutrition.gov/): Nutrition information provided by the U.S. government.
- MyPlate (https://www.choosemyplate.gov/): Healthy eating guidelines and resources from the U.S. Department of Agriculture.

Mobile Apps

- MyFitnessPal: An app that helps you track your food intake and keep a record of your physical activities.

- Yummly: An app offering thousands of healthy and personalized recipes based on your dietary preferences.

Organizations and Support Groups

- American Dietetic Association (https://www.eatright.org/): The leading organization for dietitians and nutrition professionals in the United States.
- Slow Food (https://www.slowfood.com/): A global movement promoting good, clean, and fair food.

These resources can provide you with more in-depth information on specific topics related to nutrition and real fooding.